Fantastic Thighs a

ISBN 0330 - 377...

Date:

Fantastic

Legs AND **Thighs**

MICA GRENFELL

OOKS

ADVICE TO THE READER

Before following any of the exercise or dietary advice
in this book it is recommended that you consult your
doctor if you suffer from any health problems or special
conditions or are in any doubt as to its suitability.

First published 2000 by Pan Books
an imprint of Macmillan Publishers Ltd
25 Eccleston Place, London SW1W 9NF
Oxford and Basingstoke
Associated companies throughout the world
www.macmillan.co.uk

ISBN 0 330 37740 X

1 3 5 7 9 8 6 4 2

A CIP catalogue record for this book is available
from the British Library.

Photography of Monica Grenfell by
Lesley Howling
Back cover photograph by Tony Ward,
direction by Lillie Gooch
Designed by Macmillan General Books
Design Department

Printed and bound in Belgium

Introduction

So you want a pair of fabulous legs? Well, join the club, because your bottom half is the bit of you that isn't subject to the whims of fashion. Bust and bicep size might blow with the winds of change but it's never fashionable or attractive to have massive legs. But how can you achieve the legs of your dreams when you already do every exercise ever devised, you hardly eat a thing and you're basically worn out? The answer is that you're probably doing the wrong kind of exercise and not sticking to a programme. You might still be doing the routine you did ten years ago. Well, this book is dedicated to explaining what you're doing wrong and putting you on the right track. I've included some of the most common questions I get asked and given you three workout plans to choose from. If you can commit yourself to just five or six hours a week, you'll succeed, and by the end of the book you'll have taken three major steps – you'll have saved money on classes and gym sessions that didn't work, you'll have saved time on exercise that was wrong for you and you'll be spared the psychological pressure of being constantly disappointed in how you look. So look forward with confidence. You're going to have the legs of your dreams!

Background

It's all a battle. Mother Nature wants to store fat on your hips and stomach in case you get pregnant, you want to look sleek and sexy in a pair of tight jeans. We live in ways we weren't designed for. The large, powerful muscles in your thighs, built for a life of stamina, endurance, climbing, running and walking with heavy loads, languish unused on sofas and escalators. While your fat stores are primed for survival mode you're tossing up between a treacle tart and a choc ice. Is it really any wonder that you're always hiding your legs?

Well, I use a car and a washing machine too. Life has changed but while I'm not trying to get you to hike miles in the rain just to lose half a pound, you've got to do something.

On the bright side, legs are very easy to shape. You have to get from A to B, stoop to feed the cat, and it's these sorts of movements that make the difference between gorgeous and ghastly. This book is all about how to start, which exercises are best and how to keep it up in the future. So what are you waiting for?

How It All Fits Together

We're all born with a kind of 'starter kit': a tough skeleton, internal organs and an 'overcoat' of muscles. What your muscles look like is entirely down to you and therefore it's wonderful that in theory and in practice, you really can have the shape you want by toning, stretching and almost moulding your muscles to your own specifications. The only downside is that you can't just order it up or ask someone to exercise for you – you've got to do the hard work yourself!

This is why no exercise plan is sufficient if it concentrates on individual muscle groups to the exclusion of others. If you can't do leg exercises because your knees hurt it might be down to weak, tight muscles in your buttocks or back. Exercise your whole body! If you climb stairs, muscle is the hard-working engine while fat is just a passenger.

Toning and sculpting

Traditional floorwork uses a high-rep overload, which means doing lots and lots of repetitions until the muscle you're working gets tired. You get the job done, but it takes ten times longer with ten times more effort.

Sculpting means exercising so you can do a few repetitions per set – say less than sixteen. Both improve your tone, but only sculpting can really change your shape. Sculpting uses much heavier weights with fewer repetitions – hence the term 'low-rep overload'.

What's 'overload'?

Overload sounds like serious bodybuilding but it's not. Overloading the muscle isn't dangerous and it isn't hard – it simply means working a muscle to the point where changes have to happen – and that means challenging a muscle to lift even heavier weights. Sometimes it is also called 'resistance'.

Resistance training

Resistance training is exactly what it sounds like. Imagine lifting your leg straight out in front of you – you have the weight of your leg as basic resistance but now imagine someone pushing downwards on your leg to try to stop you lifting it. This is resistance! Any movement that uses an opposing force or a weight makes the job harder, and if your muscles work harder they need more calories, their fibres grow and your shape becomes more pronounced. Some common everyday examples are sweeping, raking and vacuuming.

Stretching

I exercised for years without really stretching properly, and took my figure faults as the penalty for being short of height (5ft 2ins). Then I took up yoga and got thinner legs and hips without losing an ounce of weight! And – I was told – I looked much taller than I really am!

Here are the rules for stretching:

1 If you are not at the end of a training or workout session, warm up first by walking briskly or jogging on the spot, lightly.
2 Breathe slowly, deeply and evenly.
3 Do not stretch to the point where breathing becomes unnatural.
4 Do not overstretch.
5 Hold stretch in a comfortable position – tension subsides as it is held.

Your Questions Answered

About seven out of every ten letters I receive finish with the line 'Where am I going wrong?' It's soul-destroying to get nowhere, but exercises, like diets, need to be tailored to the individual. Here are the most common mistakes:

I've Been Exercising For A Month And I've Gained Weight! Muscle is about 22 per cent heavier than fat. Imagine getting hold of a lump of fat about 10cms square, weighing about 1lb. Now imagine picking up a similar sized piece of muscle. It would weigh about 1.22lbs, which means for every 5lbs of fat you have, the same space filled with muscle would weigh around 6lbs. The important thing is that your weight should consist of more lean muscle tissue than fat.

I've Been Doing This For Six Weeks And Nothing's Happening. There are several possible reasons for this. Either you just aren't working hard enough, you're still eating enough calories for your needs and therefore your body doesn't need its fat stores, or you're simply expecting too much, too soon. Remember, your growing processes all take about the same length of time – you wouldn't expect your hair to grow long again in a week if you had too much cut off it, but you'd still trust that it was growing.

I've Been Going To A Step Class, Played Tennis And Gone Hill Climbing. My Thighs Are Bigger Than Ever. You're doing the wrong kind of exercise. The muscles in the thighs are very large, and under stress they get bigger. You need to do more stretching and light, repetitious exercise with low weight resistance. *Vary your exercise routine so you don't get in a rut. Working muscles need balance and variety to keep in prime condition.*

When I Started Out I Toned Up In The First Fortnight. Now Nothing's Happened For Weeks! This is the principle of overload – walking will only produce improvements in people who previously took little or no exercise. If you are used to walking then walking won't train you – it will simply help you stay the same.

Getting Motivated

It's not hard to get motivated to start off a fitness plan. Just look in the mirror! You want to lose three inches off your hips, lift your bottom and get a waist. So you slog away night after night at the gym, lose an inch and a few pounds and the depression wears off. You've reached the 'plateau', where a bit of improvement's better than nothing, even though you haven't quite achieved what you set out for. So how do you keep yourself motivated from here? The problem starts because you forget how you felt. The panic as you got off the scales, the sinking heart as the zip stopped halfway up. *Remember why you wanted to do this!*

When you're 'too busy/stressed/harassed' for exercise . . .

1 Decide on a couple of days and times when you could exercise if push came to shove. Examples are when you're frittering time watching TV or generally fiddling about at home. I know that you've a lot of jobs to catch up on but you're probably spinning them out. Work faster!

2   Take trainers or easy shoes to work and do a twenty-minute walk in your lunch break to work up an appetite.

3   Make a decision to do one and then two tasks every week the 'old' way. Wash your car by hand, put the TV remote control in a drawer upstairs, clean all the windows. It's a start!

4   Do something! Everyone has an off-day, but don't give in and slump in a chair. Take the same time slot you reserved for your exercises and clear out a drawer, prune the roses, polish your shoes. You'll feel you've got something out of the day and your time won't have been wasted.

Losing Fat

Don't make the mistake of thinking that everything you eat must be 'worked off'. Food isn't there to be worked off, it's there to keep you breathing and working and getting from A to B. Exercise addicts who insist on 'working off' a polo mint end up with brittle bones and every infection going, and don't forget – fat-burning exercise is only appropriate if you have fat to burn! If you are slim and healthy you only need vigorous exercise a few times a week to keep your heart and circulatory system functioning, not to burn fat that isn't there. All the more reason, then, to get slim.

How To Find Out How Many Calories You Need

Multiply your weight in pounds by 0.409. Multiply this number by 24 – this will give you your resting metabolic rate, in other words the minimum number of calories you need in a day. Take in more than this, and without more exercise this is likely to be stored as fat.

So What Am I Going To Eat?

It isn't so much specific food that helps you have gorgeous legs, but the nutrients in the food. Here are two of the most important:

Calcium

We all know about calcium strengthening bones and teeth, but it has an important role to play in exercise. Stiffness, pain and irritated muscles are common reasons for people to find exercising unacceptable, but this is often caused by low calcium.

Magnesium

Low magnesium means your muscles stay stiff, tight and contracted when you are exercising, and this causes cramps and 'knots'. Magnesium helps a muscle to relax at the end of a movement and helps avoid these unpleasant and painful outcomes.

Calcium and magnesium are found in these power foods:

- Soya beans
- Yoghurt
- Salmon
- Sardines
- Almonds and brazil nuts
- Sunflower seeds
- Cheese
- Dark green vegetables
- Grapefruit
- Lemons
- Apples

A balanced diet

Breakfast Grapefruit, home-made muesli with almonds and sunflower seeds
Lunch Salmon and watercress sandwich, apple
Main meal Cauliflower cheese, live, plain yoghurt with chopped figs, dried apricots and sultanas

Coping With Cellulite

The best way to deal with cellulite is to avoid having it in the first place! Seriously, just like teeth don't rot the day you eat sweets, neither does cellulite show up straight away. It takes years to settle, so if you're currently smug about your smooth thighs, don't be. Getting rid of cellulite IS possible but it takes work and a healthy, liquid-rich diet to 'detoxify' your body. Exercise, and cut out tea, coffee, cigarettes and alcohol.

Eliminating Excess Fluids and Toxins

A lot is written about detoxifying, but your body does an efficient job without any interference from you. As long as you help by making sure your diet isn't stodgy and dry, detoxification is another way of saying that what goes in comes out as quickly as possible. Not an elegant topic, but an unhealthy system results in cellulite, spots, a bad skin and other symptoms of a poisoned and over-burdened digestion. Fasting is totally unnecessary. So are colonic irrigation and other fads that do nothing for you. Eat a diet rich in 'wet' foods like fruit, vegetables and dairy produce so that your system is constantly taking in water and getting rid of it. This is the only way to be sure of an efficient detoxifying process, and you should never need to resort to pills and potions.

DIURETIC FOODS

- Asparagus
- Celery
- Parsley

FIBROUS FOODS

- Melon
- Figs
- Peas
- Wholemeal Bread
- Grapes
- Sweetcorn
- Rice
- Strawberries
- Nuts

The Exercises

Your Muscle Structure

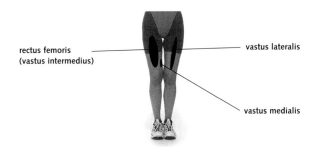

rectus femoris
(vastus intermedius)

vastus lateralis

vastus medialis

The quadriceps

The quadriceps are a group of four muscles (the rectus femoris or vastus intermedius, vastus lateralis and vastus medialis) that run down the front of your leg and their job is to straighten it. These are some of the most powerful muscles in your body and if not kept toned they become loose and short. This can lead to lower back pain and wobbly, bulky thighs that form a distinct 'bow' shape from a side view. The answer is regular toning and thorough stretching.

Quad Extensions

Always start your workout with this warm-up exercise.

1 Sit comfortably on a chair, feet flat on the floor. Now simply extend your leg out from the knee, feeling your thigh tighten. Bend and repeat.
2 Do twelve with each leg, then repeat. Always start your warm-up with this exercise. A set is twelve each leg.

Crouching Quadricep Pliés

Not the most elegant exercise, but it is one of the best! You'll really feel this after only half a dozen, but try and shake out and return to a few more.

1 With your forearms resting on a chair, lower yourself until your hips are in line with your shoulders, feet about 24ins apart.
2 Slowly raise and lower your hips, keeping your shoulders down by the chair. Do six to eight, shake out and repeat. A set is eight.

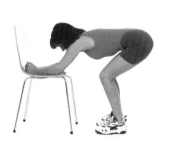
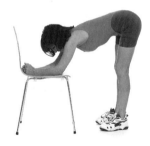

Light Quadricep Stretch

Simply stand with one leg slightly bent at the knee, and take the other foot backwards to your buttocks. Hold for twenty seconds, change legs and repeat.

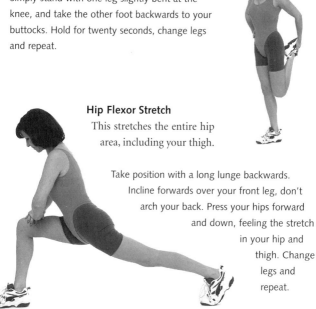

Hip Flexor Stretch

This stretches the entire hip area, including your thigh.

Take position with a long lunge backwards. Incline forwards over your front leg, don't arch your back. Press your hips forward and down, feeling the stretch in your hip and thigh. Change legs and repeat.

Strong Quadricep Stretch

1 Be sure to use a soft mat or towel. With your right hand on the floor, lean forwards enough to take the weight off your kneecap, placing your weight above the left knee instead. Here it will be better cushioned.

2 Keeping the position of the Hip Flexor Stretch, release your left hand and reach backwards for your right foot. Draw it in towards your buttocks and hold. You will feel this strong stretch at the top of your thigh. Hold for a count of twenty seconds, release a little, then repeat. Change legs and repeat.

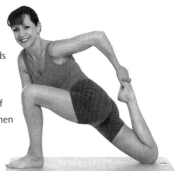

The abductors

The outer thigh muscles (the abductors) run down the outside of your thighs and are responsible for lifting your leg out to the side. Any problems with your thighs, such as the notorious 'jodphur thighs', will respond well to abductor toning.

You don't need a vast repertoire of exercises for the outer thigh – just two will do.

Abductor Lifts, Bent Knee

1 Take position lying on the floor supporting your head with one hand. Your shoulder and hip should be in a straight line, one hip directly above the other, not lying backwards. This takes the effort away from the working muscles and reduces the exercise's effectiveness.

2 Slowly lift the top leg keeping your knee facing forward. Don't jerk it up violently, and don't point your knee at the ceiling. Less is more effective. Lift twelve times. Rest and repeat. Change legs. A set is twelve each leg.

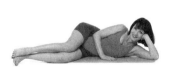 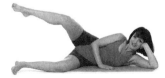

Extended Abductor Lifts

This exercise must be done very slowly; as a guide, there are about ten a minute.

1 Lie as before, but this time
   your top leg is extended, knee
   slightly bent. Your shoulder, hip and
   ankle are all in one line. Toe and knee point forwards.
2 Lift the top leg, but not so high that your hip rolls back. Go up for three
   seconds, down for three seconds. Do twelve. Change legs and repeat. A
   set is twelve each leg.

Outer thigh stretches are important to keep the muscles long and lean.

All-four Abductor Stretch

This also stretches the iliotibial band, important for runners.

Take position on hands and knees. Slowly let your
hips fall to one side, making sure your
knees stay touching. Hold for twenty
seconds. Change sides and repeat.

Advanced Abductor Stretch

This is difficult but do persevere! The stretch also incorporates the gluteal (buttock) muscles.

Lie on one side with your bottom leg straight out. Bring your top leg over with your foot on the floor and hold as near to your chest as possible. Hold for twenty seconds. Change sides and repeat.

Tip

To make your outer thighs slimmer and firmer:

- Fast cycling with little resistance, long duration
- Dancing
- Swimming – the breaststroke
- Running or jogging
- Walking
- Yoga

To increase thin outer thighs (sculpting):

- Aquarobics with weights
- Abductor lifts with light thigh weights
- Ice skating
- Horse riding

Never use heavy weights on your ankles when doing leg lifts. They can add stress to your hip joint.

The adductors

The inner thigh muscle (the adductor) runs from the groin to above the knee. Its purpose is to draw your leg in towards your body.

Standard Adductor Raises

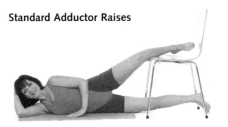

1 Lie on one side, with your top leg on a chair.
2 Slowly lift your lower leg a few inches, hold for a count of three and return to the floor. Do twelve. Rest and repeat. Change legs and repeat. A set is twelve each leg.

'Adductor Squeezes'

1 Lie on your back, putting your fists under your hips if you feel more comfortable this way. Raise both legs.

2 Keeping your feet together, bend your knees opening them outwards, pulling your feet in towards your groin. Do this slowly, twelve times. Rest and repeat. A set is twelve.

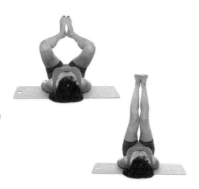

Standard Adductor Stretch

Ideal for beginners. Sit on the floor with the soles of your feet together. Lean forwards from the hip, don't bend your back. Place your elbows at the sides of your knees and press forwards to feel the stretch.

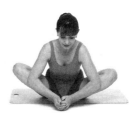

Classic Adductor and Groin Stretch

This is more difficult if you have knee problems, but it combines the groin and adductors in an effective stretch.

Lean forwards and take your weight on to your hands. Move to the side by straightening one leg and bending the other. Make sure that the foot of the straight leg remains on the floor. To increase the stretch, move the straight leg further out or bend shoulders closer to the ground. Change legs and repeat.

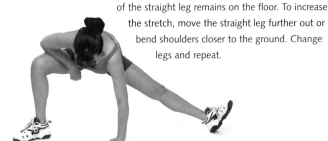

The hamstrings

The hamstrings are three muscles (biceps femoris, semi-tendinosus, semi-membranosus) that make up the backs of the legs. Exercising them gives a shapely sweep to the thighs and helps balance the quadriceps. There are two exercises that target these muscles.

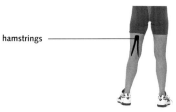

hamstrings

Hamstring Dips

1 Lie on the floor with one foot on a chair. Your other leg is extended straight up.

2 Now lift your buttocks off the floor just a few inches and feel a strong pull in your hamstrings. Release and repeat sixteen times. Change legs and repeat. Then do a further set. A set is sixteen each leg.

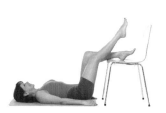
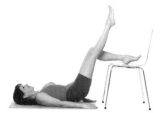

Hamstring Extensions

This exercise targets the hamstrings but also works the buttock muscles (gluteals).

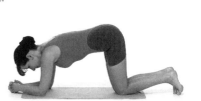

1 Lie on elbows and knees, keeping your stomach pulled in tightly. Extend one leg so it is in line with your back.

2 Lower the knee until it is nearly touching the other one then extend again. Don't fling your leg, keep control. Repeat sixteen times and change legs. Then do a further set. A set is sixteen each leg.

Hamstring Stretch Using a Chair or Table

This is the one hamstring stretch that I recommend for everyone. It takes time to master if you are new to exercise or have tight hamstrings, but it incorporates the lower back too. By using a chair or table as a support it is possible to stretch several different muscle groups at the same time.

Stand a comfortable distance from the chair and place your forearms on it. Lower the chest towards the floor. Ensure that the knees are not locked out, but straighten them as much as possible. Drop your head between your arms. Concentrate on lengthening your spine, pressing your bottom away from you and increasing the stretch in the backs of your thighs.

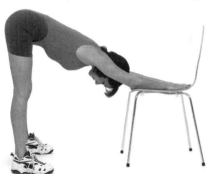

The calf muscles (gastrocnemius and soleus)

Shapely calves are the crowning glory on a great pair of legs – so don't ignore them! Shapeless calves can be easily toned and sculpted with one easy exercise, which is done two ways:

Calf Raises – Straight Leg

1 Stand on the edge of a step (your bottom stair will do, or use a telephone directory). Make sure you have something to hold on to for balance but don't lean on it. Place one foot behind the opposite calf.

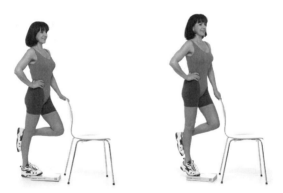

2 Raise and lower yourself slowly, allowing your heel to dip lower than the step by a few centimetres. Do eight to twelve and change legs. A set is eight each leg.

As this is a demanding exercise, you may find it difficult to do more than eight in a set. If you are trying to increase your calf size, aim to increase the number of repetitions by two a week, and the number of sets from two to thirty-two.

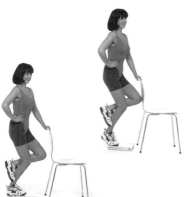

Calf Raises – Bent Leg

1 Take position as before, but this time allow a slight bend in your knee.

2 Repeat the exercise as above eight to twelve times, and change legs. Sets and repetitions as before.

Calf Stretch Against a Wall

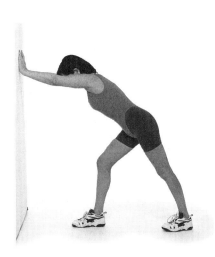

Lean with both palms flat against a wall. Place your right foot 6in from the wall and take a step backwards with your left foot. Allow your heel to press flat to the floor. Hold the stretch for twenty seconds. Now just inch your foot backwards again a few centimetres and hold again. Change feet and repeat.

Shin Stretch to Balance Calf Muscles

Crouch down as shown in the picture (opposite), kneeling on your left leg. Bring your right foot flat to the floor and place your palms flat. Lean your chest forward and keep your back straight. Keeping your right heel flat, 'walk' your fingertips out a little further. Feel the stronger stretch in the calf and shin. Hold for twenty seconds. Change legs and repeat.

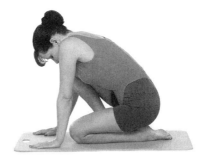

Tips

To increase the size of thin, straight calves:

Do three (twenty-four to thirty-six repetitions with rests) of Calf Raises in both positions, holding 3–5lb weights on your shoulders. Alternate with thigh exercises, coming back to repeat three sets before the end of your routine. Finish with the Calf Stretch Against a Wall. Repeat this routine for your calves on three days a week.

To slim down bulky calves:

The only way to deal with large calves is with light aerobic work as a warm-up (such as walking) followed by sustained stretching that lasts no less than ten minutes.

Exercise for All-round Fitness

A truly Fabulous Body means all of it – not just the bit you don't like! Work your legs and thighs to the exclusion of others and you risk injury from lack of muscle balance, and a weaker upper body and shape. Try to insert daily abdominal and back strengthening exercises and add swimming, a rowing machine if possible and arm exercises. Here are two exercises and a stretch to help. For the arm exercises, start with 1–3lb weights but move up to 3–5lb weights as you get fitter.

The Midriff Curl

1   Lie flat on the floor with your knees bent. Place your palms on your thighs and breathe in.

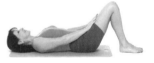

2   Breathe out as you slowly curl your neck slightly and press your spine downwards. Curl up just a few inches. Let your palms slide towards your knees. Your neck should be relaxed. Blow out rhythmically then release to the floor. You should be able to do no more than six a minute. A set is six.

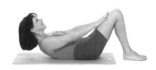

Hammer Curl

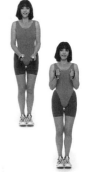

1 Stand with feet slightly apart, holding weights. Bend your knees slightly, keep your palms turned inwards and your elbows close to your body.

2 One at a time, curl each weight up towards your upper arm, stopping short of the elbow, being in a fully-bent position. (This takes the effort out of the move.)

3 Lower slowly, again being sure not to let your elbows straighten and alternate arms. Do twenty-four, rest and repeat. A set is twenty-four.

Arching Stretch

This is just one simple all-round stretch that I use for the chest and shoulder areas.

Take position on the floor, as shown. Place your hands flat behind you, fingers facing away from your body. Arch your back but not your neck. Press your ribcage upwards and away from you. Hold for thirty seconds. Release and repeat, trying to increase the stretch by taking your fingertips further away from your body. Take care! If you are new to exercise, stretch gently.

The 'Plateau'

Everybody reaches a 'plateau'. This is a sign of success because what you set out to achieve has been successful. Let me give you a good example – a daily one-hour brisk walk is excellent for your health, so if you were starting from nothing you would see a vast improvement quite quickly. Say you were a marathon-runner, though. If you had only an hour's brisk walk a day your body tone would actually get worse! *So whilst MAINTAINING a figure takes less effort than getting there, you must CHANGE the way you exercise to keep pace with your changing body shape.*

So remember:

1 Increase the EFFORT you put into exercise rather than the time spent, e.g. walk faster so you do 2 miles instead of 1½ miles in thirty minutes
2 Increase the weight you're using to challenge your muscles
3 Increase the number of sets
4 Vary your diet by introducing food you've never tried before
5 DON'T try to speed up weight loss by cutting calories even further. Stick to your three meals a day, but increase exercise.

Fitness Walking

The best exercise for all-round health, fitness and beauty. It improves circulation, loads your bones for strength, burns more calories long-term than short 'blasts' of exercise, and the daylight and fresh air help release endorphins – the feel-good hormones responsible for keeping low moods away.

1 Warm-up with 3 minutes at about 2½ m.p.h., about 90 steps per min (s.p.m.).
2 Progress to 3½ m.p.h. (120 s.p.m.).
3 Aim for 4–4½ m.p.h. (140–160 s.p.m.).
4 Lean very slightly forwards, feeling your waist 'lifting' out of your waist-band. Tighten your tummy muscles.
5 Close fists lightly and pump your arms as if walking into the wind.
6 Lengthen your neck, your spine in a straight line. Relax your shoulders.
7 Keep your feet hip-width apart. Concentrate on tightening your buttocks with each backwards step. Try to think about each stride.
8 Strike the ground with each heel purposefully. Try to take long strides, feeling as if you are 'pulling back' the ground with each step.
9 This will improve your overall shape enormously. Try to do at least 30 minutes 5 days a week, 45–60 minutes where possible.

Putting It All Together

You'll now be keen to put your plan into action, so here are three versions, one for home-based activity, one for keen and experienced exercisers using an exercise or road bike and an all-round programme, which includes upper body, swimming and treadmill or power walking. It might seem to be difficult to follow the programme at first because you will be looking at the book all the time and referring to the exercises, but you'll soon remember it. Do these plans! It's the only way to GUARANTEE success with the legs of your dreams!

Plan 1. The Quick-Fix, Anytime Home Plan

This routine is ideal for when you come home from work, while the children are playing or a quick Saturday or Sunday-morning motivator. If you have a little more time, have a twenty- to thirty-minute brisk walk.

What you need I'm assuming you have a flight of stairs, otherwise use other stairs, at your flat or at your office. Use any step for the stepping exercises.

When to do it This exercise routine is ideal for getting your workmates motivated into a pre-lunch programme.

Stair walking and running Change into loose clothing or full leotard and leggings (this might make you feel more businesslike and motivated!) and be sure to wear trainers. Walk up and down your stairs. Stair running is as it sounds. Keep up the momentum! (Sets of stair walking means up and down once, twice, etc.)

Monday

Stair exercises: four sets of walking, one set of running, repeat. Step on and off bottom stair forty times, change leg after twenty steps

FLOORWORK:

One set of Calf Raises – Straight Leg (p.28)

One set of Quad Extensions (p.17)

One set of Hamstring Dips (p.25)

Two sets of Crouching Quadricep Pliés (p.16)

One set of Hamstring Extensions (p.26)

Stair exercises: four sets of walking, two sets of running

FLOORWORK:

One set of Calf Raises – Bent Leg (p.29)

Calf Stretch Against a Wall (p.30)

Shin Stretch to Balance Calf Muscles (p.30)

One set of Abductor Lifts, Bent Knee (p.19)

One set of Extended Abductor Lifts (p.20)

One set of Standard Adductor Raises (p.22)

One set of Adductor Squeezes (p.23)

One set of Hamstring Dips (p.25)

All-four Abductor Stretch (p.20)

Advanced Abductor Stretch (p.21)

Standard Adductor Stretch (p.22)

Classic Adductor and Groin Stretch
(p.24)

Light Quadricep Stretch (p.17)

Hip Flexor Stretch (p.17)

Strong Quadricep Stretch (p.18) (if
you feel able)

Calf Stretch Against a Wall (p.30)

Shin Stretch to Balance Calf Muscles
(p.30)

Tuesday

30-minute fitness walk

FLOORWORK:

One set of Midriff Curls
(p.32)

Two sets of Hammer Curls (p.33)

Wednesday

Rest, but have a thirty- to forty-five-
minute light fitness walk

Thursday

Stair exercises: two sets of walking,
two sets of running, two sets of
walking, three sets of running

FLOORWORK:

Two sets of Calf Raises – Straight
Leg (p.28)

Two sets of Quad Extensions (p.15)

Two sets of Crouching Quadricep
Pliés (p.16)

Stair exercises: two sets of walking,
four sets of running

Floorwork:

Two sets of Calf Raises – Bent Leg
(p.29)

One set of of Abductor Lifts – Bent
Knee (p.19)

One set of Extended Abductor Lifts
(p.20)
Two sets of Standard Adductor
Raises (p.22)
One set of Adductor Squeezes
(p.23)
Stretches, as end of Monday

Friday
Thirty-minute fitness walk
FLOORWORK:
Two sets of Midriff Curls
(p.32)
Two sets of Hammer Curls (p.33)

Saturday
Complete rest

Sunday
*Try to spend longer today on a
comprehensive workout.*
Aerobics video or cycle ride, forty-
five minutes minimum
Thirty-minute brisk walk
FLOORWORK:
Two sets of Quad Extensions (p.15)
Three sets of Crouching Quadricep
Pliés (p.16), rest after each set
One set of Hamstring Dips (p.25)
One set of Hamstring Extensions
(p.26)
Two sets of Standard Adductor
Raises (p.22)
One set of Adductor Squeezes (p.23)
Stretches, as end of Monday

**Time for the week: approximately
one hour**

Plan 2. Routine For The Committed Exerciser, Using An Exercise Or Road Bicycle

This routine is suitable for all levels, but if you are an absolute beginner you might want to cycle easily at first, and leave out the hill climbs and racing sections. Keep to a warm-up and the floor exercises though, and graduate to the full routine after about three to six weeks. It will help if you also have my other books in this series, *Beautiful Bottom, Best Bust, Arms and Back*, and *Marvellous Midriff*.

Monday

CYCLING: five-minute warm-up, ten minutes in higher gear, ten-minute hill climb, five-minute easy ride

FLOORWORK:

Three sets of Midriff Curls (p.32)

Arching Stretch (p.35)

Hip Flexor Stretch (p.17)

Calf Stretch Against a Wall (p.30)

Shin Stretch to Balance Calf Muscles (p.30)

Hamstring Stretch Using a Chair or Table (p.27)

Time: forty minutes

Tuesday

CYCLING: five-minute warm-up, ten minutes in higher gear, ten-minute hill climb, ten-minute easy ride

FLOORWORK:

Light Quadricep Stretch (p.17)

Calf Stretch Against a Wall (p.30)

Shin Stretch to Balance Calf Muscles
(p.30)

Two sets of Abductor Lifts, Bent
Knee (p.19)

Two sets of Extended Abductor Lifts
(p.20)

One set of Standard Adductor Raises
(p.22)

One set of Adductor Squeezes (p.23)

Five sets of Midriff Curls (p.32)

All stretches (p.17, p.18, p.21, p.23,
p.24, p.27, p.30, p.35)

Time: one hour

Wednesday

Rest, but have a thirty-minute walk

Thursday

One-hour moderate cycle

FLOORWORK:

As Tuesday from Light Quadricep
Stretch to Adductor Squeezes
and all stretches

Time: one hour twenty minutes

Friday

As Monday

Saturday

As Tuesday

Sunday

Rest, but have a thirty-minute walk

Total time for the week:
five hours forty minutes

Plan 3. Combination Workout Using Cycling, Swimming And Home Exercise

Remember what I said about overload (p.5)? When you reach Week 3 think about increasing the intensity by adding 1lb ankle weights for your Abductor and Adductor Lifts and Hamstring Extensions, but not for Adductor Squeezes or Quad Extensions. You can hold weights in your hands for Calf Raises (3–5lbs) and add a 3–5lb weight to your hips when doing Hamstring Dips.

	Week 1	Week 2	Week 3	Week 4
Monday	(Cycling)	(Cycling)	(Cycling)	(Cycling)
	5-min warm up	5-min warm up	5-min warm up	5-min warm up
	10 mins higher gear	10 mins higher gear	10 mins higher gear	10 mins higher gear
	10 mins hill climb	15 mins hill climb	15 mins hill climb	10 mins hill climb
	5 mins cool down	5 mins cool down	5 mins cool down	5 mins cool down
	Calf Stretch Against a Wall	Calf Stretch Against a Wall	Calf Stretch Against a Wall	Calf Stretch Against a Wall

	All-four Abductor Stretch	All-four Abductor Stretch	All-four Abductor Stretch	All-four Abductor Stretch
	Hip Flexor Stretch	Hip Flexor Stretch	Hip Flexor Stretch	Hip Flexor Stretch
	Strong Quadricep Stretch	Strong Quadricep Stretch	Strong Quadricep Stretch	Strong Quadricep Stretch
	4 x 8 Crouching Quadricep Pliés	4 x 8 Crouching Quadricep Pliés	4 x 8 Crouching Quadricep Pliés	4 x 8 Crouching Quadricep Pliés
	2 x 16 Hamstring Extensions	2 x 16 Hamstring Extensions	2 x 16 Hamstring Extensions	4 x 16 Hamstring Extensions
	12 Adductor Squeezes	12 Adductor Squeezes	24 Adductor Squeezes	24 Adductor Squeezes
	3 x 6 Midriff Curls	3 x 6 Midriff Curls	5 x 6 Midriff Curls	5 x 6 Midriff Curls
	Repeat stretches	Repeat stretches	Repeat stretches	Repeat stretches
	50 mins	**55 mins**	**1 hour**	**1 hour**

Tuesday	30-min swim	30-min swim	30-min swim	30-min swim
	Classic Adductor and Groin Stretch	Classic Adductor and Groin Stretch	Classic Adductor and Groin Stretch	Classic Adductor and Groin Stretch
	Hip Flexor Stretch	Hip Flexor Stretch	Hip Flexor Stretch	Hip Flexor Stretch
	Hamstring Stretch Using a Chair or Table	Hamstring Stretch Using a Chair or Table	Hamstring Stretch Using a Chair or Table	Hamstring Stretch Using a Chair or Table
Time	**35 mins**	**45 mins**	**50 mins**	**1 hour 5 mins**

Wednesday	(treadmill)	(treadmill)	(treadmill)	(treadmill)
	3 mins 2½ m.p.h. 20 mins 4 m.p.h. 7 mins 3 m.p.h.	3 mins 2½ m.p.h. 30 mins 4 m.p.h. 7 mins 3 m.p.h.	3 mins 2½ m.p.h. 35 mins 4 m.p.h. 7 mins 3 m.p.h.	3 mins 2½ m.p.h. 45 mins 4 m.p.h. 12 mins 3 m.p.h.
	All leg stretches	All leg stretches	All leg stretches	All leg stretches
Time	**35 mins**	**35 mins**	**35 mins**	**35 mins**

Thursday	45-min cycle	45-min cycle	50-min cycle	1 hour cycle
	2 x stair walking	2 x stair walking	2 x stair walking	3 x stair walking
	2 x stair running	3 x stair running	3 x stair running	100 skips
	Calf Stretch Against a Wall	Calf Stretch Against a Wall	Calf Stretch Against a Wall	Calf Stretch Against a Wall
	2 x 8 Crouching Quadricep Pliés	2 x 8 Crouching Quadricep Pliés	3 x 8 Crouching Quadricep Pliés	4 x 8 Crouching Quadricep Pliés
	2 x 16 Hamstring Dips	2 x 16 Hamstring Dips	4 x 16 Hamstring Dips	4 x 16 Hamstring Dips
	2 x 12 Standard Adductor Raises	2 x 12 Standard Adductor Raises	2 x 12 Standard Adductor Raises	4 x 12 Standard Adductor Raises
	5 x 6 Midriff Curls	5 x 6 Midriff Curls	5 x 6 Midriff Curls	5 x 6 Midriff Curls
	15-min upper body stretch	15-min upper body stretch	15-min upper body stretch	15-min upper body stretch
Time	**1 hour 15 mins**	**1 hour 20 mins**	**1 hour 30 mins**	**1 hour 35 mins**

Friday	45-min walk or exercise video	45-min walk or exercise video	45-min walk or exercise video	45-min walk or exercise video
	Floorwork as Monday	Floorwork as Monday	Floorwork as Monday	Floorwork as Monday
Time	1 hour 5 mins	1 hour 5 mins	1 hour 5 mins	1 hour 5 mins

Saturday	As Monday	As Monday	As Monday	As Monday

Sunday	Complete rest	Complete rest	Complete rest	Complete rest

Total time for the week	5 hours 10 mins	5 hours 30 mins	6 hours	6 hours 10 mins

And Finally . . .

If you're at the bottom of the pile, there's nowhere to go but up. If you're superfit, on the other hand, training is really hard work. This is the principle of overload – walking only produces results in people who took hardly any exercise before, but if you're used to walking you won't see any changes in your body.

Improvements disappear over a few weeks, but don't let this put you off! Presumably you'll have achieved a lot but the thing to remember is that you can't put all that exercise in the bank. Give it up and you'll be back where you started in no time, but it's not all depressing. Improvements are maintained easily. A short, sharp burst of intense exercise and (especially) weights will maintain those gorgeous legs. A thirty-minute hard bike ride three times a week will do the trick. Get where you want to be first, then it's no more trouble than washing your hair. Remember what you wanted. You've made it – and you're brilliant!

MONICA GRENFELL is the *News of the World* Diet and Fitness Expert, read by millions. Her flat-stomach diet *Five Days to a Flatter Stomach*, her beauty diet plan *Fabulous in a Fortnight* and the sensational *Get Back Into Your Jeans Diet* (with its accompanying video) have all been runaway successes. All of Monica Grenfell's books are available from your local bookshop, or by sending a cheque or postal order as detailed below. Ask for details of her latest!

FABULOUS IN A FORTNIGHT
0 330 35368 3 £7.99 pb

5 DAYS TO A FLATTER STOMACH
0 7522 2130 2 £4.99 pb

THE GET BACK INTO YOUR JEANS DIET
0 330 37303 X £4.99 pb

MONICA'S FABULOUS BODY PLANS
Beautiful Bottom
0 330 37743 4 £2.99 pb
Best Bust, Arms and Back
0 330 37741 8 £2.99 pb
Fantastic Legs and Thighs
0 330 37740 X £2.99 pb
Marvellous Midriff
0 330 37742 6 £2.99 pb

Book Services By Post
PO Box 29
Douglas
Isle of Man IM99 1BQ

Credit card hotline 01624 675137.
Postage and packing free.